Introduction of Book

Are you tired of starting a fitness journey only to give up halfway through? Do you struggle to maintain motivation and see results? The key to unlocking your fitness potential lies not only in physical exertion but in mastering your mindset. In this book, you will discover seven powerful mindset hacks that will revolutionize the way you approach fitness and help you achieve lasting success.

Chapter 1: The Power of Visualization

Quote: "The power of imagination makes us infinite." - John Muir

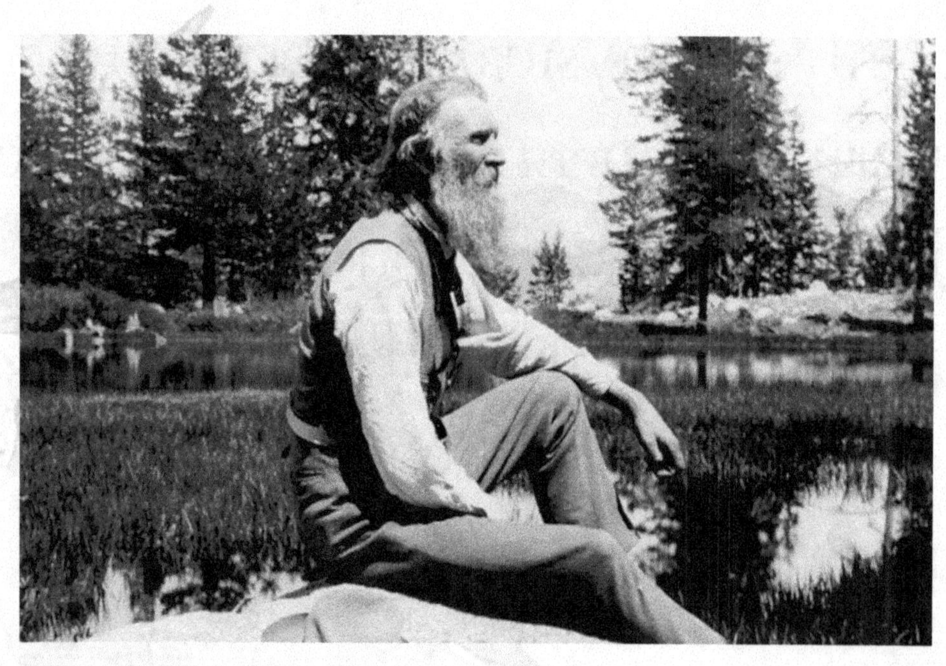

Introduction

In this chapter, we will delve into the transformative power of visualization and its profound impact on achieving your fitness goals. Visualization is not just about daydreaming; it's a powerful mental tool that can propel you towards success in your fitness journey.

Section 1: Introduction to Visualization Techniques for Fitness Success Visualization is the practice of mentally creating images or scenarios to simulate experiences. In the context of fitness, visualization involves imagining yourself accomplishing your fitness goals with clarity and detail. By vividly visualizing your desired outcomes, you can effectively program your mind for success.

Section 2: Exercises to Help Readers Visualize Their Fitness Goals Let's engage in some practical exercises to harness the power of visualization for your fitness journey:

Exercise 1: Define Your Goals – Take a moment to clarify your fitness goals. Are you striving to lose weight, build muscle, or improve endurance?

Exercise 2: Create Your Mental Movie – Close your eyes and visualize yourself achieving your fitness goals. Picture yourself with your desired physique, feeling strong, confident, and energized.

Exercise 3: Engage Your Senses – Enrich your visualization by incorporating sensory details. Imagine the sights, sounds, smells, and sensations associated with your fitness success.

Exercise 4: Feel the Emotions – Tap into the emotions of accomplishment, pride, and satisfaction as you visualize reaching your fitness milestones.

Section 3: How Visualization Rewires the Brain for Success Visualization is more than just wishful thinking; it has a profound impact on the brain. Research has shown that when you visualize yourself performing an action, the same neural pathways are activated as when you physically engage in that activity. This rewiring of the brain primes you for success by enhancing motivation, focus, and performance.

Chapter 2 : Goal Setting and Accountability

Quote: "A goal properly set is halfway reached." – Zig Ziglar

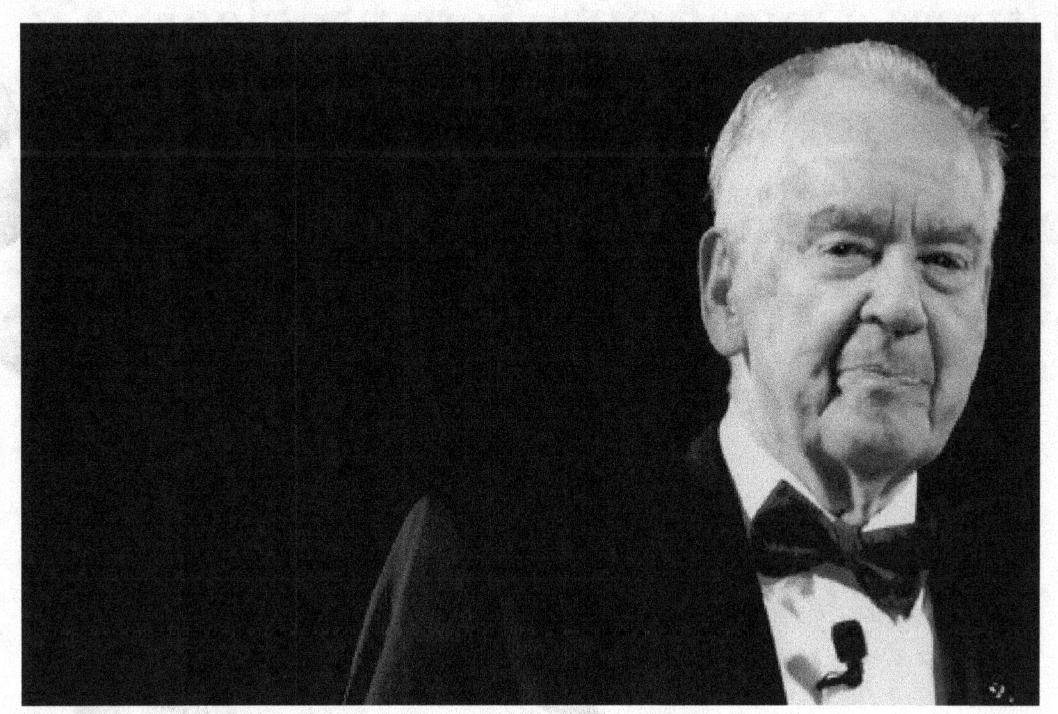

Introduction

In this chapter, we'll explore the critical role that goal setting and accountability play in achieving your fitness aspirations. Setting clear, actionable goals and holding yourself accountable are essential components of a successful fitness journey.

Section 1: The Importance of Setting SMART Goals for Fitness Effective goal setting is the foundation of any successful fitness plan. By setting Specific, Measurable, Achievable, Relevant, and Time-bound (SMART) goals, you can provide yourself with a clear roadmap for success.

- Specific: Define your fitness objectives with precision. What do you want to achieve, and why is it important to you?

- Measurable: Establish concrete criteria for measuring your progress. How will you know when you've reached your goal?
- Achievable: Set goals that are challenging yet realistic. Consider your current fitness level, resources, and timeframe.
- Relevant: Ensure that your goals align with your overarching fitness aspirations and values.
- Time-bound: Set deadlines to create a sense of urgency and focus.

- **Section 2**: Strategies for Staying Accountable to Your Goals Accountability is the glue that holds your fitness goals together. Here are some strategies to help you stay on track:

- Share Your Goals: Share your goals with a trusted friend, family member, or fitness coach. Accountability partners can offer support, encouragement, and accountability.

- Track Your Progress: Keep track of your workouts, nutrition, and progress towards your goals. Use a fitness journal, mobile app, or wearable device to monitor your performance.
- Set Milestones: Break your overarching fitness goals into smaller, manageable milestones.
- Set Milestones: Break your overarching fitness goals into smaller, manageable milestones. Celebrate your achievements along the way to maintain motivation and momentum.

- Reflect and Adjust: Regularly evaluate your progress and adjust your approach as needed. Be flexible and willing to pivot if you encounter obstacles or setbacks.

Section 3: How to Break Down Big Goals into Manageable Steps Big goals can feel overwhelming, but breaking them down into smaller, bite-sized steps can make them more manageable and achievable. Here's how:

- Identify Your End Goal: Start by clarifying your ultimate fitness objective.

- Break It Down: Divide your big goal into smaller, actionable steps or milestones.

- Prioritize: Determine which tasks are most critical and focus on completing them first.

- Create a Plan: Develop a detailed plan outlining the specific actions you need to take to achieve each step.

- Take Consistent Action: Commit to taking consistent, focused action towards your goals every day.

Chapter 3: Overcoming Self-Limiting Beliefs

Quote: "Whether you think you can or you think you can't, you're right." – Henry Ford

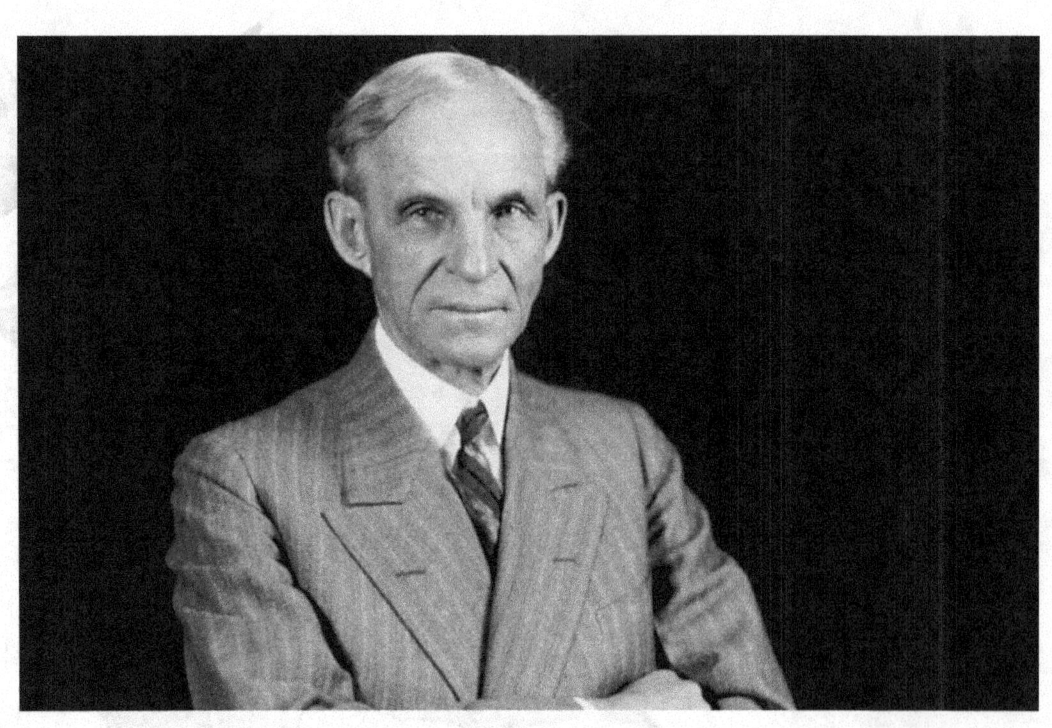

Introduction

In this chapter, we'll explore the powerful impact that self-limiting beliefs can have on your fitness journey and strategies to overcome them. Self-limiting beliefs are those negative thoughts and beliefs that hold you back from reaching your full potential. By identifying and challenging these beliefs, you can unlock new levels of success in your fitness endeavors.

Section 1: Identifying and Challenging Common Fitness-Related Self-Limiting Beliefs Self-limiting beliefs often stem from fear, past experiences, or societal conditioning. Here are some common fitness-related self-limiting beliefs to watch out for:

- "I'm not athletic enough to succeed."
- "I don't have enough time to exercise."
- "I'll never be able to reach my fitness goals."

- "I'm too old/young to get in shape."
- "I always fail at sticking to a fitness routine." Once you've identified your self-limiting beliefs, it's essential to challenge them with evidence-based reasoning and positive affirmations.

Section 2: Techniques to Reframe Negative Thoughts and Beliefs
Reframing negative thoughts and beliefs is a powerful way to shift your mindset and overcome self-limiting beliefs. Here are some techniques to help you reframe negative thinking:

- Cognitive Restructuring: Identify the irrational or distorted thoughts underlying your self-limiting beliefs and replace them with more rational, empowering ones.

- Perspective Taking: Consider alternative viewpoints or interpretations of a situation to challenge your negative beliefs.
- Gratitude Practice: Cultivate a mindset of gratitude by focusing on the positive aspects of your fitness journey and celebrating your progress, no matter how small.
- Visualization: Use visualization techniques to imagine yourself overcoming obstacles and achieving your fitness goals, reinforcing positive beliefs about your abilities.

Section 3: Building Confidence and Self-Efficacy through Positive Affirmations Positive affirmations are powerful statements that can help boost your confidence and self-efficacy. Here's how to use them effectively:

- Identify Affirmations: Choose affirmations that resonate with you and address specific areas of self-doubt or insecurity related to fitness.

- Repeat Daily: Incorporate affirmations into your daily routine by repeating them aloud or writing them down regularly.
- Believe in Yourself: Internalize your affirmations and genuinely believe in your ability to achieve your fitness goals.
- Take Action: Use affirmations as a catalyst for action, taking consistent steps towards your goals with confidence and determination.

Chapter 4: Embracing Failure and Learning from Setbacks

Quote: "Success is not final, failure is not fatal: It is the courage to continue that counts." – Winston Churchill

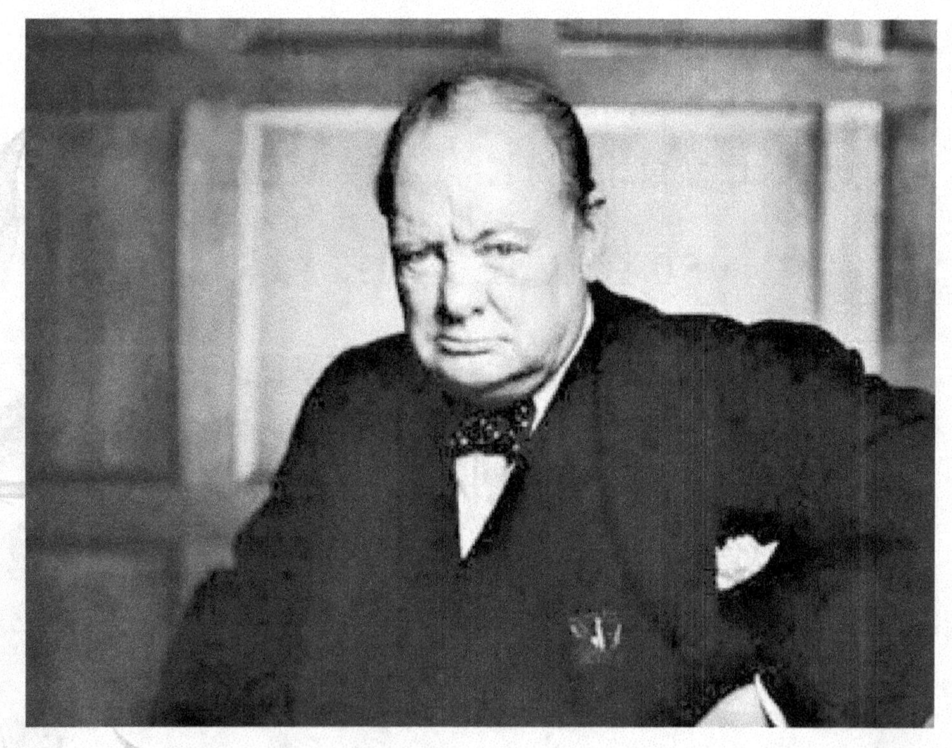

Introduction

In this chapter, we'll explore the vital role that failure and setbacks play in your fitness journey and strategies to embrace them as opportunities for growth. Failure is not the opposite of success; it's a stepping stone on the path to success. By reframing failure and learning from setbacks, you can bounce back stronger and more resilient than ever before.

Section 1: The Role of Failure in the Journey to Fitness Success Failure is an inevitable part of any worthwhile pursuit, including fitness. Instead of viewing failure as a roadblock, see it as a valuable learning experience and an opportunity for growth. Here's why failure is essential in your fitness journey:

- Failure Builds Resilience: Facing and overcoming failure strengthens your resilience muscle, making you more resilient to future challenges.

- Failure Sparks Innovation: Failure forces you to reevaluate your approach and find new, creative solutions to overcome obstacles.
- Failure Fuels Motivation: Failure can be a powerful motivator, inspiring you to work harder and smarter towards your fitness goals.

Section 2: Strategies for Reframing Failure as an Opportunity for Growth
To reframe failure as an opportunity for growth, consider the following strategies:

- Adopt a Growth Mindset: Embrace the belief that failure is not a reflection of your abilities but an opportunity to learn and improve.
- Focus on Progress, Not Perfection: Shift your focus from achieving perfection to making progress. Celebrate small victories and milestones along the way.
- Practice Self-Compassion: Be kind to yourself when you experience setbacks. Treat yourself with the same kindness and understanding you would offer a friend.

- Seek Feedback: Solicit feedback from trusted mentors, coaches, or peers to gain valuable insights and perspectives on how to improve.

Section 3: How to Bounce Back Stronger After Setbacks After experiencing a setback, it's essential to bounce back stronger than ever. Here's how:

- Analyze What Went Wrong: Take a step back and analyze the factors that contributed to the setback. Identify areas for improvement and develop a plan to address them.

- Adjust Your Approach: Use the lessons learned from the setback to refine your strategy and approach moving forward.

- Cultivate Resilience: Focus on building resilience by practicing mindfulness, gratitude, and self-care.

- Analyze What Went Wrong: Take a step back and analyze the factors that contributed to the setback. Identify areas for improvement and develop a plan to address them.
- Adjust Your Approach: Use the lessons learned from the setback to refine your strategy and approach moving forward.
- Cultivate Resilience: Focus on building resilience by practicing mindfulness, gratitude, and self-care.

- Stay Persistent: Remember that setbacks are temporary. Stay committed to your fitness goals and keep pushing forward, no matter how challenging it may seem.

Chapter 5: Cultivating a Growth Mindset

Quote: "The only limit to our realization of tomorrow will be our doubts of today." - Franklin D. Roosevelt

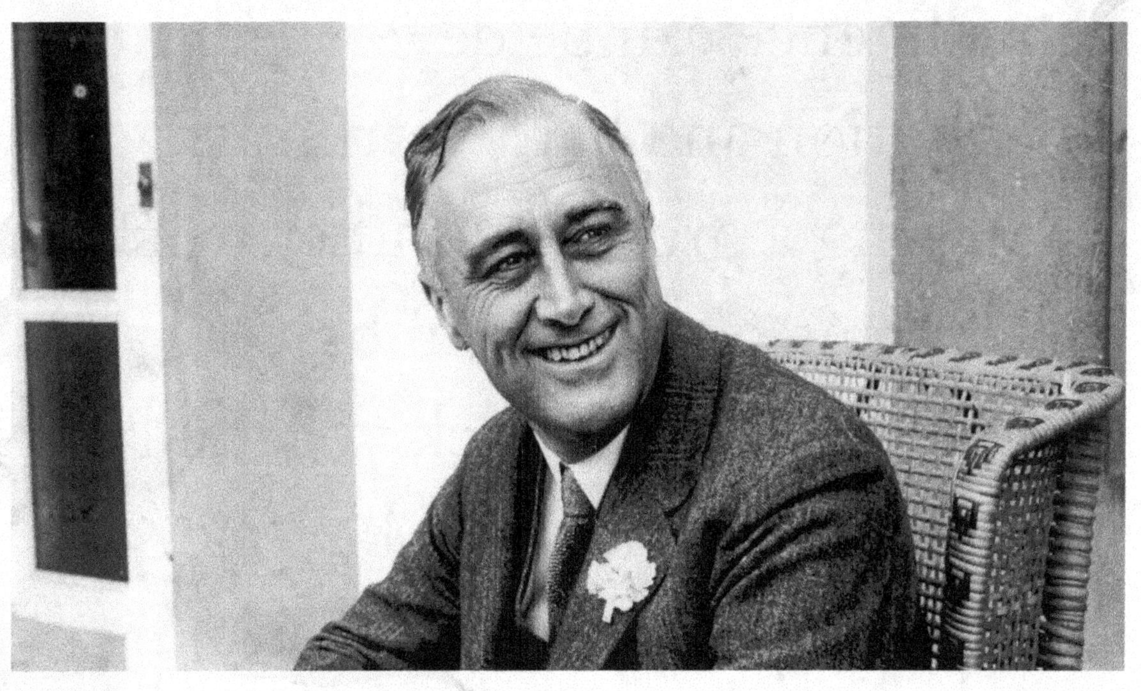

Introduction

In this chapter, we'll explore the transformative power of cultivating a growth mindset in your fitness journey. A growth mindset is the belief that your abilities and intelligence can be developed through dedication and hard work. By adopting a growth mindset, you can overcome obstacles, embrace challenges, and unlock your full potential in fitness and beyond.

Section 1: Understanding the Difference Between a Fixed and Growth Mindset In a fixed mindset, individuals believe that their abilities are fixed traits and cannot be changed. They may avoid challenges, give up easily, and view effort as fruitless. In contrast, individuals with a growth mindset believe that they can improve and grow through effort and perseverance. They embrace challenges, persist in the face of setbacks, and view failure as an opportunity for learning and growth.

Section 2: Techniques for Developing a Growth Mindset in Fitness Here are some techniques to help you cultivate a growth mindset in your fitness journey:

- Embrace the Power of Yet: Replace statements like "I can't" with "I can't yet." Recognize that your current abilities are not fixed and can be developed with time and effort.

- Focus on the Process: Shift your focus from outcomes to the process of growth and improvement. Celebrate the effort, progress, and learning that occurs along the way.
- View Challenges as Opportunities: Instead of avoiding challenges, seek them out as opportunities for growth and development. Challenge yourself to try new exercises, set ambitious goals, and step outside of your comfort zone.

- Practice Self-Reflection: Regularly reflect on your progress, setbacks, and areas for improvement. Use self-reflection as a tool for self-awareness and continuous growth.
- Surround Yourself with Growth-Minded Individuals: Surround yourself with individuals who embody a growth mindset and support your journey towards growth and development.

Section 3: Embracing Challenges and Seeking Out Opportunities for Growth Challenges are an inevitable part of any fitness journey, but they also present opportunities for growth and improvement. Here's how to embrace challenges and seek out opportunities for growth:

- Set Stretch Goals: Set ambitious but attainable goals that push you outside of your comfort zone and challenge you to grow.

- View Setbacks as Learning Opportunities: Instead of viewing setbacks as failures, see them as opportunities for learning and growth. Identify the lessons learned from setbacks and use them to inform your future actions.

- Stay Persistent: Stay persistent and resilient in the face of challenges and setbacks. Remember that growth takes time, effort, and patience.

Chapter 6: Creating a Supportive Environment

Quote: "Always surround yourself with people who are even more talented and competent than you.
" – Stephen Covey

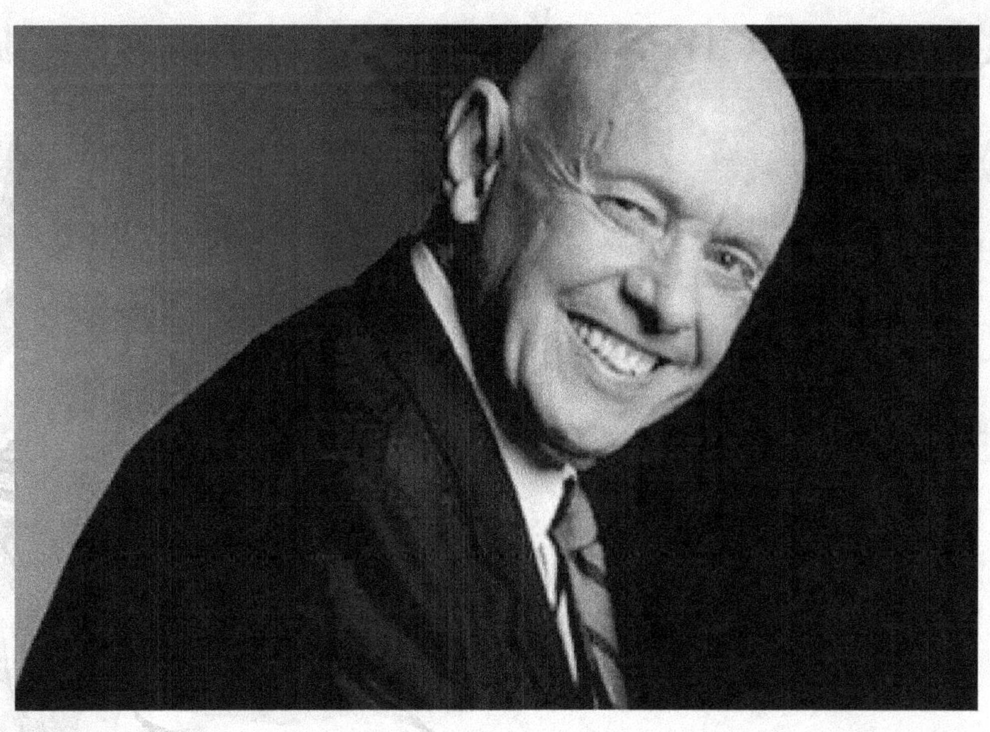

Introduction

In this chapter, we'll explore the crucial role that your environment plays in your fitness journey and strategies for creating a supportive atmosphere that fosters growth, motivation, and success. Surrounding yourself with like-minded individuals and building a supportive fitness community can make all the difference in achieving your fitness goals.

Section 1: The Importance of Surrounding Yourself with Like-Minded Individuals Your environment has a significant impact on your mindset, habits, and behaviors. Surrounding yourself with like-minded individuals who share your fitness goals and aspirations can provide invaluable support, motivation, and accountability. Here's why it's essential to surround yourself with like-minded individuals:

- Motivation and Inspiration: Being around people who are passionate about fitness can inspire and motivate you to stay committed to your goals.
- Accountability: Like-minded individuals can hold you accountable to your fitness commitments and provide encouragement during challenging times.

- Knowledge and Support: Sharing experiences, tips, and advice with others who have similar fitness goals can help you navigate challenges and obstacles more effectively.

Section 2: Strategies for Building a Supportive Fitness Community Here are some strategies for building a supportive fitness community:

- Join Fitness Groups or Classes: Participate in fitness classes, group workouts, or online communities focused on your specific interests or goals.
- Find a Workout Buddy: Partnering with a workout buddy can provide accountability, motivation, and companionship during workouts.
- Attend Events and Workshops: Attend fitness events, workshops, or seminars to connect with like-minded individuals and expand your network.

- Volunteer or Coach: Get involved in coaching or volunteering opportunities within the fitness community to give back and connect with others who share your passion.

Section 3: How to Deal with Unsupportive Friends and Family Members While surrounding yourself with supportive individuals is essential, you may encounter unsupportive friends or family members along the way. Here's how to deal with unsupportive individuals:

- **Communicate Your Needs:** Clearly communicate your fitness goals, boundaries, and needs to unsupportive friends or family members.

- **Seek Support Elsewhere:** If certain individuals in your life are consistently unsupportive, seek support from other sources, such as online communities, support groups, or professional coaches.

- Set Boundaries: Set boundaries
  with unsupportive individuals to
  protect your mental and
  emotional well-being. Surround
  yourself with people who uplift
  and encourage you on your
  fitness journey.

Quote: "Alone we can do so little;
together we can do so much." -
Helen Keller

Chapter 7: Practicing Self-Compassion and Patience

Quote: "The journey of a thousand miles begins with one step." - Lao Tzu

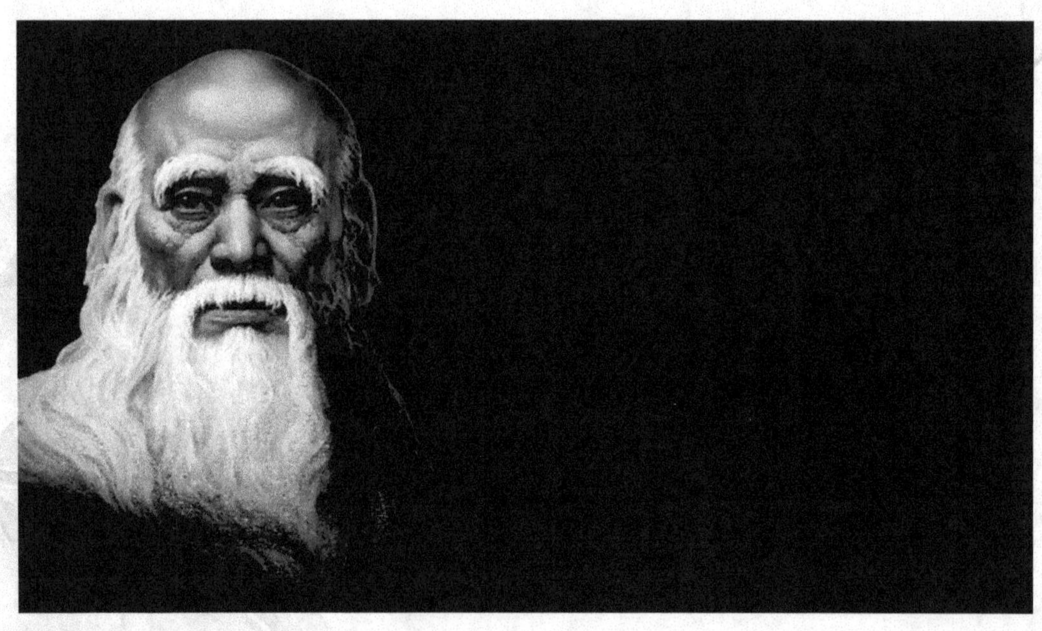

Introduction

In this chapter, we'll explore the transformative power of practicing self-compassion and patience in your fitness journey. Self-compassion is the practice of treating yourself with kindness, understanding, and acceptance, especially during challenging times. By cultivating self-compassion and embracing patience, you can navigate setbacks, overcome obstacles, and achieve long-term success in your fitness endeavors.

Section 1: Why Self-Compassion is Essential for Long-Term Fitness Success Self-compassion is essential for several reasons:

- Resilience: Self-compassion fosters resilience by helping you bounce back from setbacks and challenges with greater ease and grace.
- Motivation: When you treat yourself with kindness and understanding, you're more likely to stay motivated and committed to your fitness goals.

- Emotional Well-being: Practicing self-compassion improves your emotional well-being by reducing stress, anxiety, and negative self-talk.

Section 2: Techniques for Practicing Self-Compassion During Setbacks and Challenges Here are some techniques for practicing self-compassion during setbacks and challenges:

- Self-Kindness: Treat yourself with the same kindness and understanding you would offer to a friend facing similar challenges. Practice self-soothing and self-nurturing behaviors.
- Common Humanity: Remember that setbacks and challenges are a natural part of the human experience. You're not alone in experiencing difficulties on your fitness journey.

- Mindfulness: Cultivate mindfulness by staying present and aware of your thoughts, feelings, and sensations without judgment. Mindfulness helps you respond to setbacks with greater clarity and compassion.

- Self-Validation: Validate your own experiences and emotions without judgment or criticism. Acknowledge your efforts, progress, and strengths, even in the face of setbacks.

Section 3: The Importance of Patience and Perseverance in the Fitness Journey Patience and perseverance are essential qualities for achieving long-term success in fitness. Here's why they're important:

- Sustainable Results: Fitness is a journey, not a destination. Sustainable results take time, consistency, and patience to achieve.

- Learning and Growth: Setbacks and challenges are opportunities for learning and growth. Embrace the journey, celebrate progress, and stay committed to your goals.
- Mental Resilience: Patience and perseverance build mental resilience, enabling you to stay focused, motivated, and determined in the face of adversity.

In The End

Congratulations on completing
"7 Mindset Hacks for Fitness Success!"
May your journey be filled
with self-compassion, patience,
and triumph.